LAW OF ATTRACTION

HOW TO DRAW MORE HAPPINESS, HEALTH AND SUCCESS INTO YOUR LIFE IN THE FUTURE THROUGH VISUALIZATION & AFFIRMATIONS.

JEREMY S. MEYER

CHAPTER ONE

LAW OF ATTRACTION

How to draw more happiness, health and success into your life
in the future through visualization & affirmations.

Incl. practical tips for every day

Jeremy S. Meyer.

MS MEDIA

1st edition 2019

CHAPTER TWO

Table of Contents:

- Foreword / Introduction
- The Law of Attraction - A Natural Law
- The law of attraction - Origin
- Known Formulations for the Law of Attraction
- The law of attraction in psychology
- The law of attraction and its manifestations
- The first characteristic - the attraction
- The second characteristic - the exclusion principle
- The Law of Attraction in the Past and Present
- The law of attraction and its effect
- Positive and negative thoughts
- Conscious and Unconscious
- Why the law of attraction is subject to multiplication
- Why the start of the day is crucial
- What the manifestation is all about
- How to put the law of attraction into practice
- The law of attraction and creative process
- How you can influence the law of attraction itself

CHAPTER THREE

Foreword / Introduction

Even though physics lessons in school might not have been your thing, you can't get around different laws. I'm sure you've heard of the law of attraction before. This physical law of nature, whose theory is many centuries old, often serves as a motif for various films or forms the basis of an interesting book. But also in everyday life you will encounter this regularity from time to time. I'm sure you've heard the words "opposites attract" before. But is that really the case? This question will be explored, inter alia, in this guidebook.

The law of attraction, however, has to serve much more often. That's how you invoke this law when things go really wrong in life. It is said that you attract negative things when you are not well anyway. But if you are well, then you attract all the positive energies of the universe. Again, the law of attraction takes hold.

.   .   .

This book will explore whether this law really exists beyond physics. How it affects love, for example, and how everyone can benefit authentically yet individually, are just some of the aspects that will be examined below.

The Law of Attraction - A Natural Law

Before explaining how the law of attraction affects or can affect our daily lives, we should first get to the bottom of the origin of this lawfulness. Actually, it can also be described as a law of nature. Because the law of attraction is a basic concept of the universe. If you put it very simply, you could say, "Same attracts same." This already shows that this law can be applied to many areas. In physics it plays a similarly decisive role as in society or psychology.

CHAPTER FIVE

The Law of Attraction: Origin

Even though the law of attraction is an ancient natural law, it did not originate in science until the end of the 19th century. Thus it is closely linked to the US-American New Thought Movement. This is a social, but also philosophical movement that can be translated into German with the term Neugeist movement.

CHAPTER SIX

KNOWN Formulations for the Law of Attraction

In order to make the terminology of this law even more comprehensible, various formulations can be used. I'm sure you've heard a lot about that.

One of the most common formulations that are often mentioned in this context is the term "adiposity":

- Same attracts same
- Equal and equal like to be joined
- To us happens according to our faith
- As one calls into the forest, so it echoes out again.
- You'll be what you think of the most.
- You're not wearing what you want.
- You put on what you think is true.
- I consciously influence whom or what I pay attention to.

These different formulations, either known as wisdom or proverb, written in the Bible or by various scientists and writers, make it clear that the law of attraction is not a mystery. Rather, we have this legality in our own hands.

CHAPTER SEVEN

THE LAW of attraction in psychology

If you take a look at the website of a provider of life counselling, it quickly becomes clear that the law of attraction is frequently applied, especially in psychology. It's about bringing the inside and the outside together. The inside is your thoughts and feelings. These in turn have a direct effect on what you experience, i.e. the outside. The important thing now is to link the two. The interior is also always determined by the personal and individual attitude to life. So if you approach something with the right attitude, you'll also get along better with the external influences. Both can't be done without each other. How dependent their own feelings and thoughts are on external appearance factors, however, is seldom realized by many people. So you may also like to consider the law of attraction as a real helper in everyday life. It supports you in getting things into context and can even lead to more satisfaction and a more positive attitude towards life in the end.

CHAPTER EIGHT

THE LAW of attraction and its manifestations

In order to illustrate how often you are confronted with the law of attraction in your everyday life, it also helps to deal with the basic manifestations. Thus, the law of attraction is based on two essential characteristics, attraction and exclusion. On the one hand, it is based on the principle of equal oscillation. This almost magically attracts things and people. However, the law of attraction also says that you can only attract what you are occupied with. For example, if you have no resonance for things you are not interested in, they will hardly influence your world of feelings and thoughts, and you cannot magically attract these things either.

CHAPTER NINE

THE FIRST CHARACTERISTIC - the attraction

In order for the law of attraction to have any effect at all, it needs foundations. These are formed by your thoughts and feelings. It doesn't matter whether you consciously or unconsciously think or feel something. These things, thoughts and feelings are what you deal with. So you automatically attract external factors that deal with the same topic - at least that's the theoretical basis. You're thinking of something in particular. The more intensely you think about it, the higher the attraction for the exterior, which is directly connected with the felt or the thought.

CHAPTER TEN

THE SECOND CHARACTERISTIC - the exclusion principle

For things which are important to us and which we consider to
be true, we form, as science says, a resonance body. So in a way,
we're opening up to it. The outside world of a human being is
therefore not made up exclusively of the things around him.
Rather, only those things for which there is a resonance within
are perceived particularly intensively.

CHAPTER ELEVEN

THE LAW of Attraction in the Past and Present

The law of attraction has been occupied by many different people for many centuries. It was expressed in some form in writings, in stories, but also in music and paintings. But the law of attraction is also found in all world religions. That again speaks for the fact that it really is always there, no matter what you believe in, no matter which picture you look at, no matter which exciting book you are reading or which song you are listening to.

The scientist Rhonda Byrne even found out that the law of attraction was an issue even in antiquity. It was carved in stone 3000 BC. The various historical and social epochs then ensured that the law of attraction was further spread. It was above all teachers who created stories to explain the course of life and thus also this regularity. However, people from earlier centuries or millennia have expressed themselves differently than we do today. This has led to people today not understanding these messages and perceiving them as encrypted. Perhaps this is one reason why so few people really consciously apply the law of attraction in their lives.

It is not only thanks to the fact that historians analyse and decipher the ancient writings that the law of attraction has become famous. It is above all the outstanding film "The Secret" from the early 2000s that brings us closer to the law of attraction. The centuries probably had to pass. It was first necessary to create forms of representation that would help to convey the function and effectiveness of the law.

CHAPTER TWELVE

THE LAW of attraction and its effect

Have you now become curious how the law of attraction actually works? Then first make yourself aware of one thing: The law of attraction always works, there is no stop button and it never pauses in terms of its effectiveness. So as soon as you start thinking about something, the law of attraction is automatically activated. It doesn't matter whether you think of something good or something less good. It also doesn't matter in which time you are mentally on the move. One can think of the past, deal with the present or dare a look into the future. The law of attraction is always there.

The law of attraction is not only continuous. It also affects all aspects of human existence. It can affect interpersonal relationships as well as your health. The themes of money and work can also be directly affected by this magical attraction. So it can be said that the law of attraction influences every moment of your life. It is a manifestation of your feelings and thoughts.

It should also be noted, however, that the law of attraction is by no means a product of chance. Thus the reaction to thought and felt is not random. Rather, this law functions as precisely as a clockwork. In the introduction to this book we talked about the fact that the law of attraction is often perceived individually. One thinks, for example, that one attracts negative things and experiences particularly strongly if one already thinks negatively anyway. This is true, but the law of attraction does not affect one person more than another. The law of attraction unfolds its effect in the same way all over the world. It can hit every single one equally hard. You can only determine the intensity of the effect yourself. If you deal very intensively with a topic and know how to transform thoughts into certain feelings, then the effect will of course be much more intense. So for the law of attraction it is completely irrelevant who you are and where you are at home.

CHAPTER THIRTEEN

Positive and negative **thoughts**

Every person thinks sometimes of something positive and some-times of something negative. However, the law of attraction is completely indifferent to this in terms of its effect. For it to be activated, it doesn't matter whether you're thinking about the last beautiful summer vacation or the painful separation from your partner. The law of attraction is only interested in how intensely you think a thought. No matter whether it's positive or negative in nature. That is why what was written here in the introduction is also true. If, for example, you belong to those people who often think of something negative, then you will certainly also magically attract negative experiences more frequently. If, on the other hand, you are a person who thinks predominantly positively, then it is predominantly the positive circumstances that will accompany you in your life. Actually, the law of attraction is as simple as it is ingenious. So you can always assume that you're right. The law of attraction is as neutral as the universe itself. The universe is there, but it doesn't evaluate

the things around it. Rather, it is the person who values. Therefore it is up to you how you evaluate your thoughts, feelings or
certain experiences. If you see it positively, you also attract all
the positive situations that come with it. But if you think negatively, happiness is a long way off. So it is always up to you how
the law of attraction affects you and your life.

CHAPTER FOURTEEN

Conscious and Unconscious

Since the law of attraction is not only neutral, but leaves it up to the thinking and feeling person, that is you, whether something is viewed positively or negatively, it does not matter whether you send out your thoughts and feelings consciously or unconsciously. You might think the previous remarks are now fictional nonsense. But the law of attraction doesn't care at all about that either. It always works whether you believe in it or not, whether you understand it or not.

It is also certain, however, that one can make better use of this legality in any case if one believes in it. Most people hardly think about whether they think consciously or unconsciously. That is why the law of attraction often only unconsciously applies to most people. It has an effect, but is not necessarily perceived consciously. But you'll get a lot more out of it if you start making this law your own. When you begin to think more consciously, then you perceive more consciously, then you also live more consciously. Only then will you understand the way this law works and be able to enrich your daily life.

There are certainly different ways for you to start thinking more consciously. Meditation, for example, is just one way that can help you get to know your thoughts and control them a little better. You should also always say to yourself: "I am master of my thoughts". At some point these words pass into your own thinking and feeling and make you aware of many things that were hidden in the unconscious part of your world of thoughts until now.

CHAPTER FIFTEEN

WHY THE LAW of attraction is subject to multiplication

There are truly many ways to scientifically substantiate the law of attraction. Thus one can also use a mathematical assumption. The law of attraction is subject to the factor of multiplication so that it can show its full effect. If one tries to reduce this mathematical formula to a simple denominator, then it can be said that a certain thought always attracts thoughts of the same kind. A positive thought inevitably triggers many more positive thoughts.

Of course, this multiplication also works in the other direction. Thus a negative thought is also attracted by further negative thoughts. Not only your thoughts but also your feelings are subject to the same kind of multiplication. So a positive thought will bring many more positive thoughts and will also make you feel good or even better. A negative thought on the other hand

influences your feelings in the negative direction, you will probably feel worse.

CHAPTER SIXTEEN

Why the start of the day is crucial

Thoughts and feelings only develop further in the course of a day. However, it is the start of the day that has a decisive influence on our world of feelings and thoughts. So if you go into a new morning with a good feeling and positive thoughts, you will also think positively and feel good during the course of the day. However, it is very easy to get into a negative emotional vortex in the morning. When you wake up and think, "I don't feel like going to work today" or "I don't really want to get up at all", it's melancholy thoughts that accompany you. These can then run like a red thread through your whole day.

So why should you spoil your own day when you are burdened with negative thoughts? Rather, you should think of something positive right after waking up. For example, it helps if you become aware in the morning of what things you are actually grateful for. This gratitude often leads to beautiful thoughts or memories of the people with whom one associates this gratitude. So the start of the day was a success. In the morning you can also think about what things and experiences you can look forward to during the day. So living the law of attraction also means initiating a chain reaction. Of course you should limit yourself to the positive direction. After getting up think of something beautiful and in the course of the day many positive thoughts and feelings will follow.

CHAPTER SEVENTEEN

WHAT THE MANIFESTATION is all about

But to live by the law of attraction also means to control manifestation. So some time will always pass before thoughts become
feelings and then external events and experiences. So if you find
that you are thinking a negative thought, then you should use
the following time to transform that negative thought into a
positive one. With this you manifest what you have just thought,
make it conscious and change it to your own advantage.

CHAPTER EIGHTEEN

How to put the law of attraction into practice

Everyone has bigger goals. Every person also has different dreams, which he would like to realize at some point. The more often you think of your unfulfilled wishes and dreams, the more conscious they become to you. So you bring these dreams straight into your life. You are more often concerned with what can in the end also lead to a successful implementation.

To keep this up, you can stick to a simple belief, as already described in the book and film "The Secret". "Thoughts become things." Thought becomes tangible. Wishes become reality. What you experience in your life, you influence to a large extent yourself. So if you learn to control your thoughts and steer them in the right direction, then you learn at the same time how to pursue and achieve your goals.

. . .

The law of attraction acts like an invisible helper who is always there. Hopelessness could therefore quickly become a thing of the past. Of course, there will always be situations in life where you have to start anew. Maybe you were thinking positively, but the result wasn't the same as your imagination. Then perhaps the strategy needs to be changed. The great thing about it, however, is that the law of attraction also makes a difference. Then there are new approaches, new thoughts and new feelings that you can orientate yourself on. These thoughts and feelings attract further thoughts and feelings and cause positive events.

CHAPTER NINETEEN

THE LAW of attraction and creative process

Furthermore, the law of attraction or its application is based on the principle of the creative process. There are three principles you should be aware of. Then it will also be easy for you to consciously apply the law of attraction. Enquiry, belief and reception are the three key words that help you to consciously juggle your thoughts.

CHAPTER TWENTY

How you can influence the law of attraction itself

To quickly integrate the law of attraction into your life, you can follow two simple but basic rules. First of all you should pay close attention to your thoughts and the words associated with them. On this point the law of attraction is particularly thorough and precise. The more you think a thought, if you think it to the end and express the thought correctly, the faster the multiplication works and the law of attraction unfolds its full effect by attracting more positive thoughts.

You can also easily influence the pace of your life with the law of attraction. Don't think a thought because it just has to be thought. Think a thought because you want to think it. Here, the more passionately you think of something, the more consciously you draw it into your life.

CHAPTER TWENTY-ONE

WHY THE LAW of attraction is lived so little

Now you have experienced how much power you can gain over your thoughts and feelings and thus also over what happens in your life. You have learned how positively you too can benefit from the law of attraction. Nevertheless, one can rightly ask oneself the question why not everyone lives according to this simple law, when it is so simple. This question can be answered with the so-called Will-not epidemic.

This means that although people think a lot, most people actually think predominantly of something negative rather than something positive. Then the law of attraction can work, because it flows in both directions, but of course it cannot have the desired effect on the fulfillment of wishes or dreams. It's somehow incredible, but for centuries many people have been thinking and saying what they actually don't want. You could also say that you can hardly stand in your own way anymore.

. . .

The law of attraction still works, of course. It manifests what you thought, whether you wanted it or not. If one wants to justify this assumption, then one can make use of psychology. So the subconscious is responsible for this phenomenon. According to various psychological studies, the human subconscious assumes that exactly what we deal with mentally and emotionally should enter our lives. Nevertheless, we cannot tell our brain what to do and what not to do. Rather, one must try to make clear to one's subconscious what one really wants and not what one does not want.

CHAPTER TWENTY-TWO

Certainly the subconscious belongs to those things which cannot be influenced 100% by man. However, you can test the reactivity of your subconscious with a small test. This will tell you how you actually think and whether you are already affected by the Will-Non-Epidemic. You could say to yourself, "There's no pink elephant behind me right now." Of course it is clear that there is no pink elephant there either. But still, when you spoke those words, you had the image of a pink elephant in front of your eyes. But you wanted to achieve exactly the opposite, namely to find out that there is no pink elephant behind you. The way you've just seen the picture of the pink elephant, your subconscious is constantly going through it. It can't know whether you want something or not, whether something is causing you grief or trouble. At least not on his own and just like that. The subconscious here is like the universe. It takes in and accepts the messages, but it does not interpret them, only you do so with the power of your thoughts.

CHAPTER TWENTY-THREE

FIRST EXAMPLE

UNDERSTANDING the Subconscious - Some Examples

To reconcile the subconscious and the law of attraction, a few practical examples are given. On the one hand, a thought is assumed. The second point is how the law of attraction can receive the thought words. Third, you can also see what you could say and think instead so that the law of attraction works for you in the right way.

First example:

You say or think, "There's no way I want to be late."

What the law of attraction makes of it, "I want to be late."

What you should think instead is, "I'm definitely on time."

. . .

Explanation:

If you are exclusively concerned with the idea of coming too late, you are not really thinking precisely. There's no real, fixed goal behind your thought. Also, the words "I don't want to be late" imply a touch of indifference. If you now consciously control and steer your thoughts and tell yourself that you will definitely reach your destination on time, then you have a fixed goal. You automatically think in the direction that you will be punctual and that gives you a more positive feeling than the fact of doubting it. It is therefore fundamentally a matter of making a fact out of an original intention, out of a simple expression of will. To create a path that one consciously perceives and follows just as consciously. First intellectually and then outside of one's own world of thoughts.

CHAPTER TWENTY-FOUR

SECOND EXAMPLE

Second example:

You say or think, "I don't want to catch a cold."

What the law of attraction makes of it is, "I'm gonna catch a cold."

What you should think instead is, "I am and I feel healthy."

Explanation:

In the beginning there is the fear that you think you might get a cold. You don't want it, but you are so preoccupied with it that your subconscious only perceives "cold" or "cold". But not the fact of whether you want to catch a cold or not. But at the moment when you have this fear, you are probably healthy and there is actually no reason at all to fear becoming ill now. So be aware of how you feel right now. Of course you can still get a cold, but you don't conjure it up by wasting too many thoughts on it unnecessarily.

CHAPTER TWENTY-FIVE

THIRD EXAMPLE

Third example:

You say or think, "There's no way I want to fight."

What the law of attraction makes of it: "I want to argue much more."

What you should think instead is, "Everything around me is harmonious."

Explanation:

You may be thinking about a recent disagreement with an important person. Of course, a difference of opinion can always lead to an argument. You are aware yourself that you want to put this difference of opinion aside and think that you don't want a quarrel. Your subconscious doesn't realize it, though. It only hears "fight" and not that you don't really want a fight. But if a dispute has not yet broken out, then it is up to you to make sure that it stays that way. You can make sure that the existing harmony is preserved. That the difference of opinion is cleared out of the way and that it does not come even to a quarrel.

CHAPTER TWENTY-SIX

Sensibly perceiving and using feelings

Now you may be wondering if you really need to monitor and control all your thoughts now. That would certainly be helpful, but let me tell you that this is simply impossible. Clever minds have once discovered that a single person thinks up to 60,000 different thoughts a day. These cannot be monitored and controlled. For one thing, the day is too short. On the other hand, you'd probably be smoking your head fast. There's still an easier way to bring order to your thoughts. Now it's about your feelings. Feelings are triggered by your thoughts. If you not only consciously perceive your thoughts, but also proceed in the same way with the resulting feelings, then you will learn more about your thoughts. A feeling triggers something in you, it always lets you know what you're thinking.

CHAPTER TWENTY-SEVEN

INTERACTING with the environment

It's not just your own thoughts and feelings that make the law of attraction work, by the way. It also works in conversations with your environment. For example, if someone tells you something negative, it will unfortunately have a negative effect on your thoughts. Instead, you should try to lead the conversation in a positive direction. If this is not possible, it also helps to turn away from this conversation. That's the only way you can stop a negative thought pull. Just always tell yourself that the negative thoughts are the weak thoughts and that the positive thoughts stand for strength. Just try to think good thoughts. This certainly does not work immediately and not always. But in any case you learn to think more positively and you can radiate this to others as well.

CHAPTER TWENTY-EIGHT

THE LAW of attraction from the point of view of mutual influence

Even if you may want it sometimes, you do not have the power to intervene directly in another person's life. This may be the case with external factors. Thoughts and feelings, however, are always reserved for yourself. Conversely, this of course means that no one else can create anything in your life. The formation of one's own life is always subject to one's own self.

However, this does not mean that mutual interference is excluded. But for this you have to be on the same wavelength with your opponent. For example, if you want a friend to think more positively, then your friend must open up to your words. If he does not consider them credible, then the mutual influence will not work. Of course, you should only try to influence another person in a positive way, because after all, the law of attraction says that influencing can only be good for yourself.

Sender and receiver of information must therefore always go hand in hand so that a positive influence can be exerted.

CHAPTER TWENTY-NINE

How do you feel about others?

I'm sure you also think about other people around you. There will be people whom you admire and about whom you think only positively. But there will also be people in your environment who you think less of and about whom you think negatively. However, be aware that your thoughts about others have no influence on others. If you think negatively about a person, it won't hurt him. You, on the other hand, could be harmed by these negative thoughts. Make yourself aware that you are hurting yourself by letting negative thoughts about others into your life. Many people think more about other people than about themselves. But this also means that they run away from their own thoughts and feelings and try to repress them. It is always more convenient to deal with the things of others than perhaps with one's own problems or desires. But you won't make any progress like this. The other must think for himself as well as it is your task to think for yourself. However, this principle naturally does not only apply to negative thoughts. If you think of another person with admiration, he may rejoice, but it does not change him. However, this thought could already make you feel positive.

CHAPTER THIRTY

THE LAW of attraction in love

The law of attraction works always and everywhere. However, there is one force that can strongly influence the effect. So it can be assumed that the law of attraction works above all in love. With your thoughts you can attract other people. The law of attraction is actually the reason why people love each other and why they become aware of each other at all. People who love each other have their differences, but love arises from many similarities. There are points of attraction that allow two people to open up to each other and, if they are doing well, to resonate with each other in a vibrating and uniform way. If this happens to you, then the law of attraction has unfolded its full effect.

CHAPTER THIRTY-ONE

ARE opposites really attracted to each other?

Now that we have become acquainted with the law of attraction, the question remains as to the myth. Thus it is always spoken of that opposites should attract each other. Whether in physics or in life. But is that really the case? After all, the law of attraction says that like is attracted by like. According to this, opposites should not actually attract each other.

In physics, different poles always attract each other. But can this be applied to interpersonal relationships? And if so, how long can this go well, if you take the assumption that people and thoughts with equal voices attract each other as a basis?

CHAPTER THIRTY-TWO

A STUDY that examined the contrasts

In the recent past, there have been numerous studies that have examined whether opposites in society and in love actually attract each other or whether they are just a myth. If it's a myth, the law of attraction would be right. The study was conducted in 2016 by Cornell University. 900 people between the ages of 18 and 24 took part. However, before the question of opposites was examined, the test persons were first asked what was important to them at all when choosing a partner. First of all, it was examined to what extent the individual personality structure and distinct personal characteristics play a central role in the search for a partner. To make it easier for respondents to answer this question, they were given ten different traits that might play a role in finding a partner. These should then be ranked by the study participants according to their importance. The participants then had to relate the same properties to themselves and assign them accordingly. The character traits available for selection were divided into four main areas for better classification.

These areas certainly play a role when choosing a partner. The interviewees had to assess how important the financial and social position of their partner is to them. Sexual fidelity was also listed in terms of its importance as a trait of character. Further criteria were family awareness and the external appearance of the potential partner.

CHAPTER THIRTY-THREE

Results of the study

If we now look at the first results of the study, it can already be said that the law of attraction probably takes effect more frequently than the fact that opposites may attract each other after all. Those people who saw themselves as particularly attractive and successful in the survey also proceeded in the same way when choosing a partner. For them, these characteristics were more important than for the respondents, who did not have a particularly high opinion of themselves. This would prove, or at least support, that the same thing attracts rather than the opposite. The professors who conducted this study at Cornell University also came to the same conclusion. It is true for Western society that people feel attracted to commonalities. It was only in a few exceptional cases that the opposites gained the upper hand.

CHAPTER THIRTY-FOUR

HOW THE LAW of attraction can work - A few tips

These many theoretical pages on the law of attraction will be followed by some practical tips. It may be that you have read the previous chapters attentively, but now you find that the law of attraction, or rather its implementation in your life, simply does not work. However, since the law of attraction always works, you can be sure that it will work for you. The following seven tips are designed to help you see more clearly and find approaches and ways to successfully apply this law in your life.

However, before you are given the tips, you should know one more thing. The law of attraction is only one of several principles of creation. Of course it always works, but you can only use it correctly if you know the other principles of creation. Only when all these components are brought into harmony does the law of attraction work in your life just as it should.

· · ·

To make a pictorial comparison, you can now go to the time

the day you took your driving test. There you had to pay attention to many things at the same time. You had to learn how to
use the car's gas pedal. But also clutch, gearshift and brake had
to be known. Besides, you had to flash at the right time and then
watch out for the forest of signs that surrounded you. Admit-
tedly, that's a lot of things at once. If you apply the driving test
now to the law of attraction, then the law is merely the accelerator pedal of your car. But if you can use the accelerator, you still
don't know how the brake works. This example is just to show
you that one cannot do without the other. And that the law of
attraction functions only when it is harmoniously associated
with all other principles of creation or with the other laws of life.

Tɪᴘ 1: Get to know the principles of creation

The seven creation principles of human life date back to the time of the ancient Egyptians. There they were passed on as the so-called Hermetic Laws. Of course, the seven principles of creation are a very special topic, to which one could dedicate an entire ebook. Therefore, they should only be mentioned here. But online you will find enough sources to get to know the other six essential life principles better.

These are the seven principles of creation:

- The Principle of Spirituality
- The principle of resonance / attraction
- The principle of vibration
- The principle of polarity
- The Rhythm Principle
- The principle of cause and effect

- The principle of creation

- The names of these principles will help you to
  understand why they should be called together with the
  law of attraction. In many cases, the one also requires
  the other. If you make yourself aware of this, you also
  gain easier control over your thoughts.

- Tip 2: Let the law of attraction work for you

As I mentioned before, you're supposed to have wishes and dreams. You should think positively about them and believe that you can reach them. But you also have to consider the reverse conclusion. However, not all dreams come true in the course of a lifetime. Whether you are to blame for this yourself or whether external factors are responsible for it, is at this point left open. If wishes cannot be fulfilled and dreams cannot be turned into reality, then you should still have positive thoughts. Only in this way can the law of attraction take effect as desired. Just tell yourself you're still happy. Enjoy what you have. Think about whether you really need what you want. Set realistic goals, and you'll feel even more satisfied when you achieve them. It is just as important as having goals and realising wishes to appreciate the existing value. So it's about being at peace with yourself. This is the only way to think positively about something. And only in this way is it ultimately possible to make new goals and wishes a reality. So you should learn and also be prepared to let go of some wishes. Then you should still learn to be satisfied, even if perhaps not everything you dream of is fulfilled.

TIP 3: Wishes arise on different levels of creation

In order to really apply the law of attraction, you must be aware of your desires. Wishes have a deeper meaning and do not just arise out of a whim. It is scientifically assumed that desires always arise at a certain level of creation. Science divides the levels of creation into three different areas. On the one hand there is the level of creation of the body. This includes all things that arise on your physical level. The second level of creation is the level of thought. This includes various emotions and everything that you can grasp with your mind. For the law of attraction, however, the third level of creation is the most important. This is the plane of the soul. This level contains the other two levels of creation. So it is the overall construct from which you can derive your wishes. If, for example, you want to reach a goal, what you want from your heart or what your soul really wants, then it is much easier for you to reach it.

. . .

And exactly at this point all aspects that have already been mentioned to the law of attraction apply. You create a wish out of passion and out of your soul. In this way you build up a positive basic relationship with him, which is also reflected positively in your thoughts and feelings and ultimately in your actions. If, on the other hand, you want to create something that does not lie deep in the soul, it will also be much more difficult for you. You can also imagine the law of attraction in connection with the three levels of creation of desires, thoughts and feelings as a great musical work. You can imagine the level of the soul as a composer. So your soul is responsible for the music of your life. She determines what's really important to you and what's not.

THEN THERE IS the level of creation of the mind, of thoughts and feelings that you can understand as a conductor. The conductor decides how the composition of your soul should be interpreted and played. So this level helps you to make decisions, to steer your life and thoughts and actions exactly into the channels you want to steer them into.

The third level of creation, i.e. the physical level, is then the orchestra that performs the composed piece. All physical components must harmonize with each other. Speaking of the orchestra, the instruments must be well tuned and able to work harmoniously with each other. So that they can perform the piece of your soul the way you want it to be and have determined it together with your mind, the conductor.

TIP 4: Question your own decision

Making decisions is part of everyday life. However, we often only think that we have actually made a decision. Therefore, you should always review and question your decisions thoroughly. Of course, with this you also check the awareness of your thoughts. Here you must find out whether the thought you are working on at the moment is a wish or whether it has already become a goal. As stated in the practical examples, you must make an expression of will a fact. Wishes are daring and unspecific. They're something you think about. They also ensure that the Law of Attraction provides you with many valuable approaches that will lead you in the right direction.

However, the cycle is not yet complete here. A wish must become a goal. So your wish cannot be fulfilled by positive thinking alone. Only when the desire has become the goal will you work on it and make it a reality. Then the initial positive thoughts become goals and methods, which in the end hold positive life events in store for you. However, a wish should always be checked. Not every wish is really a goal in the end. So you should always ask yourself if this is really your wish that comes from the heart. So you should consider carefully whether you want to make your wish the goal. Only then is this decision for further action to be made.

Tɪᴘ 5: Always ask the question why

Since the law of attraction is a chain reaction, you have to think from the beginning. So you should always be aware of what is behind a wish, a thought or a goal. So you're always wondering why. You will find out whether these thoughts, wishes and goals can really have a positive influence on your life. If you discover in the course of answering these questions that there is actually no deeper meaning behind it, you should rather deal with really important things in order not to stand in your own way.

If, for example, you wish yourself a money blessing, then ask yourself why you actually want or need to be rich. Often someone who wants to be rich just doesn't want to be as poor as he is at the moment. All he really wants is for the current situation to change. Often this is then projected onto material things, like a lot of money. However, you'd better be aware of your present situation. Question why you are not satisfied, or try to come clean with the topicality. Maybe you're not rich and can't buy yourself everything you want. But you have enough money to make your life pleasant. One can also be quite satisfied with that.

So check the meaning of your wishes and goals before you go about implementing them. Only when the question of why produces a meaningful answer should you think further about it. You should be satisfied with what you have. Because that also has its deeper meaning. Once one understands this, it is also easier to live with oneself and one's life in real and honest harmony. You can successfully apply the law of attraction if you tell yourself that it is okay as it is right now. At the same time, however, you may wish for a change. Perhaps it is just not the right time at the moment to turn this wish into reality.

TIP 6

Tɪᴘ 6: Find connection to your own soul

This tip is by no means meant to be an excursion into esotericism or deeper religious studies. But you can't completely avoid these things if you want to apply the law of attraction. The esoteric would now say to you that you should make contact with your higher self. That can be God or the Creator. However, this is not about esotericism. That's why you should always make sure that you stay in touch with your soul.

Thoughts and feelings belong together and favour each other. If a feeling arises in you that is not really anchored in your heart or soul, then you will notice this from your thoughts. You waste valuable thoughts when you give yourself to feelings that you don't actually feel. Which you may only feel because it was caused by some situation, another person, or an external condition. But they don't come from inside you. Then those thoughts or feelings aren't worth much to you. So always stay with yourself. Stand by what is and what you want to change or wish for. But don't try to please someone else or to feel something, because you should feel it the same way.

The law of attraction also applies in these cases, but not necessarily advantageously. Once you have landed on a wrong track with thousands and thousands of thoughts and feelings, it is usually very difficult to get back on the right track, the best one for yourself.

Tɪᴘ 7: Beliefs and esteem

At the beginning of this guide a proverb was already mentioned. "As it calls into the forest, so it calls out again." There's no better way to describe the law of attraction. Beliefs and objectives should therefore coincide. For example, if you wish to be loved, then of course it doesn't work because you simply wish to be loved. It also doesn't work if you can't value yourself. You can only experience love if you also have a good attitude towards yourself, if you can also love yourself. So it doesn't work if you want to feel more love on the one hand, but on the other hand you think I can't do anything anyway. These two assumptions are completely contradictory. But the law of attraction says that like is attracted to like. Therefore, your beliefs should always fit the goals and desires you set for yourself.

CHAPTER THIRTY-FIVE

The Law of Attraction: A Conclusion

Basically, it can be said that the law of attraction is a positive thing - and not just because it is based on positive thought. In contrast to all the laws that you got to know during your physics lessons, this is finally a law that you can understand and apply.

That is already the next good aspect. The law of attraction works and always works, even if you don't notice it. Although you cannot influence its existence, you can control and actively influence its effects on your life.

If you want to apply the law of attraction, you have to be aware of many things. It is your thoughts that cause many more thoughts. It is all these thoughts, about 60,000 a day, that are responsible for what you feel and how you feel. And it is your thoughts and feelings that shape your goals and desires. And it is your desires and goals that lead to what actually happens in your life.

The more positive you approach something, the more positive what comes out in the end.

The more satisfied you are with yourself and this here and now, the easier it is for you to achieve future goals and turn wishes into reality.

If you want the law of attraction to work not only for yourself, but also in interaction with your environment, then stay with yourself, think positively, and look for like-minded ones, for opposites only attract in rare cases as a result of different studies.

Finally, don't forget to consider every day of your life as a gift. Even when there are gloomy days, they all have their raison d'être and their meaning. It's up to you how you stared into the day. Just pay attention to your first thought in the morning. He is the one who will influence your thoughts and feelings throughout the day. Be thankful and think of the positive things that will happen in the course of your life

of the day. The time will pass faster even on dull days and you can look forward to the positive.

Preserve positive thoughts and feelings and try to preserve them. Negative events and experiences, on the other hand, should not be viewed too negatively. Rather, you should fathom the meaning behind it and learn something from it that can work differently in the future.

· · ·

In short, it is up to you whether the law of attraction really works as it should. If it works, it will definitely affect your appeal to others. That's a positive train of thought, which I'm sure you like to follow.

ABOUT THE AUTHOR

My name is Jeremy S. Meyer. I am 49 years old and live in beautiful Lucerne in Switzerland. I was born in the USA and grew up there, in New York City, the BIG APPLE.

In my life I have experienced a lot, I was even briefly homeless once and a few years later with the rich and beautiful at eye level. Since I can think (or write), I have been working as a journalist, author and consultant for some of the most powerful companies on the planet. I left nothing out of children's books, travel reports, glossy magazines and also business news.

To be honest, there's not much I haven't written about yet.

Because of my work with people and also because of the traveling connected with it, I and my wife (thank God) got to beautiful Switzerland at some point. In the course of time, the topics of personality development, rhetoric, and the art of leading a happy, holistic life became increasingly important to me. The inner urge arose to share my knowledge with others and to enrich their lives positively.

Many of the things I have learned in my various stations I pass on to thousands of people in my books and coaching sessions today.

As a mentor, I love to inspire others and get the real potential out of you. I get my drive again and again through the wonderful stories that life writes, and to keep them is for me daily a joy and a vocation at the same time.

"Life is so much more than 9 to 5"

AND NOW TO US.... since we both got closer in the last words - almost became friends... (At least you know more about me now than about many of your FB friends) it would be great if you could support me...

In my business, I live on INTEGRATED customers and of course on their stories, so I would be very happy about a recession.

So you'd be doing me a service of friendship. ;-)

Please take these 30 seconds and appreciate the work I and my team have put into this book and into your future.

Thank you very much in advance.

.   .   .

You are also welcome to recommend me or read my other books, you can find them all on my author page.

So, that was it now also with the self-advertisement. ;-)

I thank you for your trust and wish you a wonderful life.

DISCLAIMERS

DISCLAIMERS

The content of this book has been checked and compiled with great care. However, no guarantee, liability or warranty can be assumed for the completeness, correctness and up-to-dateness of the contents. The content of this book represents the personal experience and opinion of the author and is for entertainment purposes only. The content should not be confused with medical help. No legal responsibility or liability is accepted for any damage caused by counterproductive exercise or error by the reader. No guarantee for success can be given. The author therefore assumes no responsibility for the non-achievement of the goals described in the book! If you have any questions, please read the package insert or ask your author or publisher! All the best